Nash Night Publishing

Copyright © 2023 Nash Night

Fit for Life:

The Ultimate Guide to Achieving Optimal Health and Fitness

Table of Contents:

form and technique, and offer various exercises and workouts for beginners to advanced levels.

5. Flexibility and Mobility: Discuss the importance of stretching, yoga, and other mobility exercises in improving flexibility, preventing injury, and maintaining good posture.

6. Recovery and Rest: Explain the importance of recovery and rest days, and provide tips on how to properly recover from workouts and prevent injury.

7. Motivation and Mindset: Discuss the role of motivation and mindset in achieving fitness goals, and provide tips and strategies for staying motivated and positive throughout the journey.

8. Home Workouts: Offer tips and strategies for working out at home with limited equipment, including bodyweight exercises and at-home equipment options.

9. Staying Active: Provide tips for incorporating physical activity into daily life, including ways to stay active while at work, travelling, or at home.

10. Advanced Fitness: Offer tips and strategies for advanced fitness enthusiasts, including training for a specific sport or event, bodybuilding, and powerlifting.

Chapter 1: Setting Fitness Goals

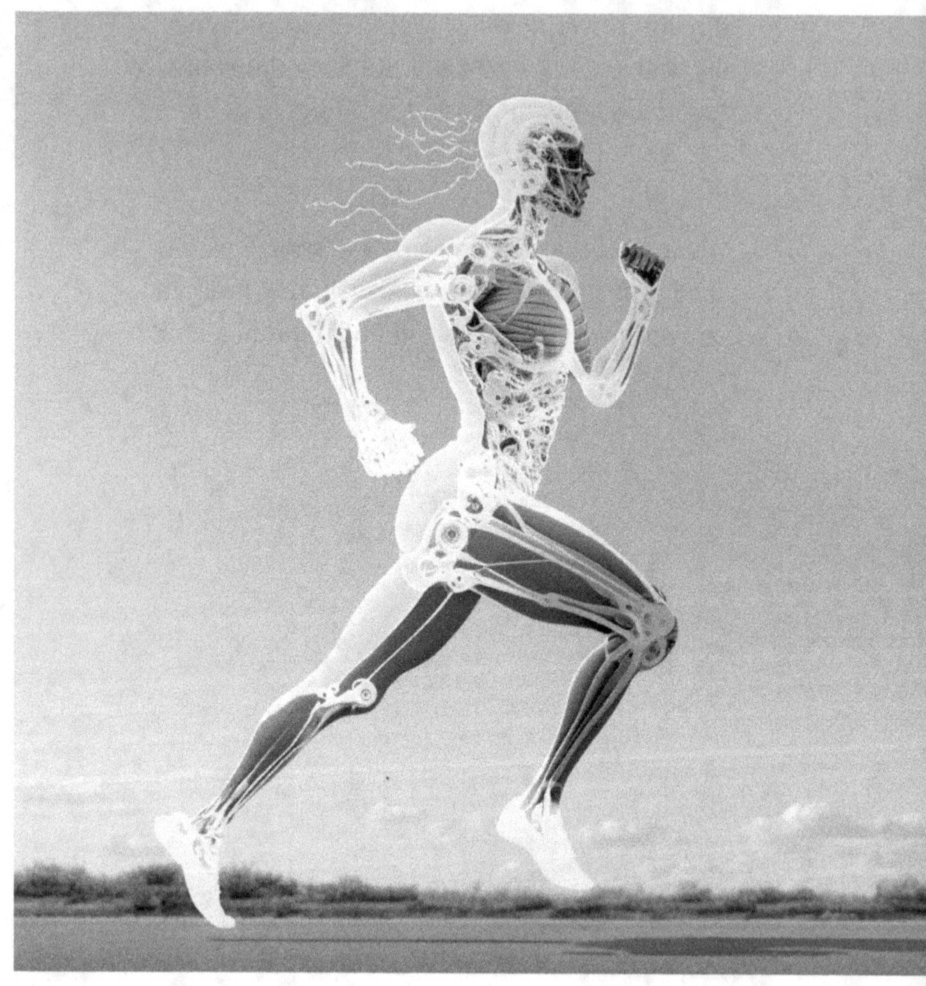

Congratulations on taking the first step towards your fitness journey! This chapter is all about setting effective and unique fitness goals that will help you achieve the healthy lifestyle you desire. The key to setting goals that work for you is to be specific, realistic, and personalised. In this chapter, we'll discuss the steps you need to take to set effective fitness goals.

Step 1: Assess Your Starting Point

Before you start setting goals, you need to have an understanding of your current fitness level. Assessing your starting point will give you a clear idea of where you stand and what you need to improve. It's essential to be honest with yourself during this step, as it will help you set realistic goals.

You can assess your fitness level in a variety of ways, including taking a fitness test, measuring your body fat percentage, or tracking your daily physical activity. Once you have a clear picture of where you stand, you can move on to the next step.

Step 2: Define Your "Why"

Understanding why you want to get fit is crucial to setting effective and unique fitness goals. Your "why" should be specific to you and should motivate you to stick to your goals. It could be anything from wanting to feel more confident in your body to improving your overall health.

Take some time to reflect on your "why" and write it down. This will help you stay motivated and remind you of why you started in the first place.

Step 3: Set Specific Goals

Now that you have a clear idea of your starting point and your "why," it's time to set specific goals. The key to setting effective goals is to make them specific, measurable, achievable, realistic, and time-bound.

For example, instead of setting a general goal like "get fit," you could set a specific goal to run a 5k in six weeks or to do 20 push-ups without stopping. These goals are measurable, achievable, and time-bound, which makes it easier to track your progress and stay motivated.

Step 4: Create a Plan

Once you have your goals in place, it's time to create a plan to achieve them. Your plan should include a workout schedule, nutrition plan, and any other activities that will help you achieve your goals. It's essential to make your plan unique to you, taking into consideration your lifestyle, preferences, and limitations.

For example, if you're someone who enjoys outdoor activities, you could plan to go hiking or biking a few times a week. If you're someone who prefers to work out at home, you could create a home workout routine using free weights or bodyweight exercises.

It's also important to break your goals down into smaller, achievable steps. This will help you track your progress and stay motivated. For example, if your goal is to run a 5k in six weeks, you could start by running for 10 minutes a day and gradually increase your running time.

Step 5: Track Your Progress

Tracking your progress is crucial to staying motivated and making sure you're on track to achieve your goals. There are many ways to track your progress, including keeping a fitness journal, using a fitness app, or taking progress photos.

It's important to celebrate your progress along the way, no matter how small. Recognizing your achievements will help you stay motivated and committed to your goals.

In conclusion, setting effective and unique fitness goals is essential to achieving a healthy lifestyle. Take the time to assess your starting point, define your "why," set specific goals, create a personalised plan, and track your progress. With dedication and consistency, you can achieve the healthy lifestyle you desire.

Chapter 2: Nutrition for Fitness

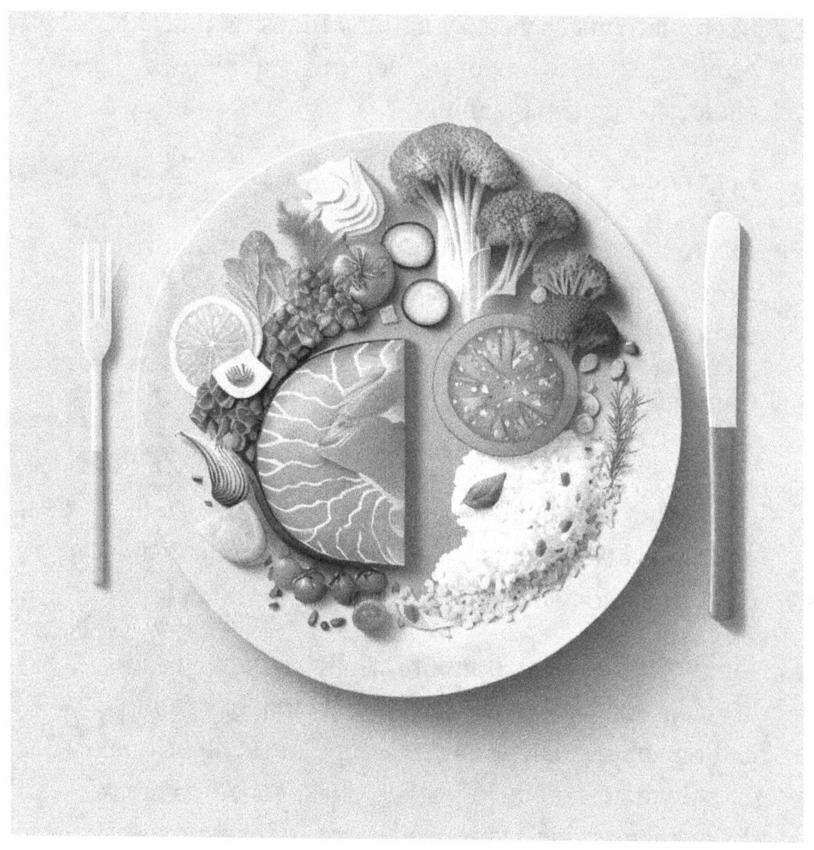

Nutrition plays a crucial role in achieving and maintaining optimal fitness and health. In this chapter, we'll detail the essential macronutrients and micronutrients needed for optimal fitness and health, provide guidance on portion control, healthy food choices, and meal planning.

Macronutrients

Macronutrients are the three main nutrients required in large amounts in the human diet. These nutrients are carbohydrates, protein, and fat.

Carbohydrates

Carbohydrates are the primary source of energy for the body. They are found in foods like fruits, vegetables, grains, and dairy products. Carbohydrates can be further classified into two categories: simple and complex.

Simple carbohydrates are broken down quickly and provide a quick source of energy. Examples of simple carbohydrates include sugar, honey, and syrup. Complex carbohydrates, on the other hand, take longer to break down and provide a sustained source of energy. Examples of complex carbohydrates include whole grains, beans, and vegetables.

Protein

Protein is essential for building and repairing tissues in the body. It's also important for maintaining a healthy immune system and producing hormones and enzymes. Good sources of protein include meat, fish, poultry, beans, and nuts.

Fat

Fat is another macronutrient that is essential for optimal health. It helps with the absorption of vitamins and minerals, provides energy, and helps regulate body temperature. Good sources of healthy fats include nuts, seeds, olive oil, and avocados.

Micronutrients

Micronutrients are essential vitamins and minerals that are required in smaller amounts in the human diet. While they may be required in smaller amounts, they are no less important than macronutrients.

Vitamins

Vitamins are organic compounds that are required for various biological processes in the body. They can be found in fruits, vegetables, and other foods. Some essential vitamins include vitamin C, vitamin D, and vitamin B12.

Minerals

Minerals are inorganic compounds that are also essential for optimal health. They can be found in foods like nuts, seeds, and leafy greens. Some essential minerals include calcium, iron, and magnesium.

Guidance on Portion Control, Healthy Food Choices, and Meal Planning

When it comes to nutrition for fitness, portion control and healthy food choices are crucial. It's essential to choose nutrient-dense foods that provide the necessary vitamins and minerals your body needs to function optimally. Some healthy food choices include lean protein sources, fruits, vegetables, whole grains, and healthy fats.

Meal planning can also be a helpful tool in ensuring that you're meeting your nutritional needs. When planning meals, it's important to consider the macronutrient and micronutrient content of the foods you're consuming. A balanced meal should include a serving of lean protein, a serving of complex carbohydrates, and a serving of healthy fats.

In terms of portion control, it's important to be mindful of the amount of food you're consuming. Use a food scale or measuring cups to ensure that you're consuming the appropriate serving size. Eating slowly and mindfully can also help with portion control by allowing you to recognize when you're full.

Conclusion

In conclusion, nutrition plays a critical role in achieving and maintaining optimal fitness and health. It's essential to consume a balanced diet that includes macronutrients like carbohydrates, protein, and fat, as well as micronutrients like vitamins and minerals. Choosing nutrient-dense foods, practising portion control, and meal planning can all be helpful strategies in ensuring that you're meeting your nutritional needs

Chapter 3: Cardiovascular Fitness

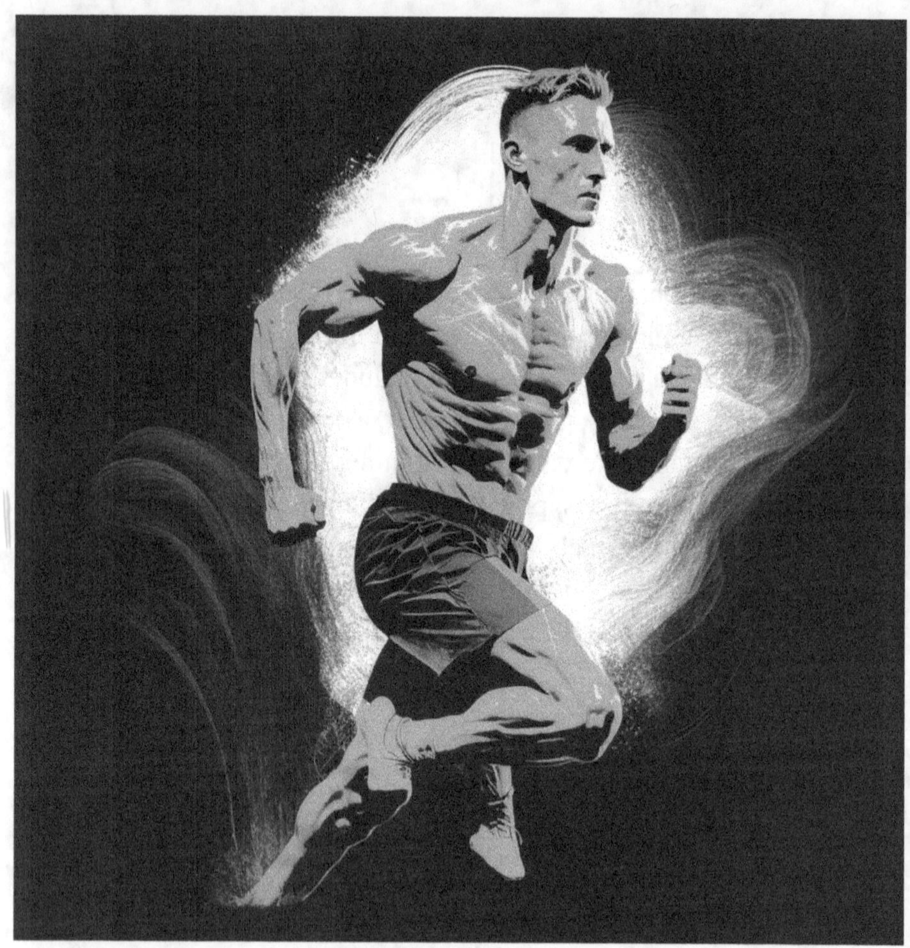

In this chapter, we'll discuss the importance of cardiovascular health and provide different types of cardio workouts that readers can incorporate into their fitness routine.

Importance of Cardiovascular Health

Cardiovascular health refers to the health of the heart and blood vessels. It's essential for optimal health and fitness because it helps improve endurance, stamina, and overall cardiovascular function.

Engaging in regular cardiovascular exercise has been shown to have numerous health benefits, including:

Lowering blood pressure

Reducing the risk of heart disease and stroke

Improving lung function

Reducing the risk of type 2 diabetes

Improving overall cardiovascular function

Types of Cardio Workouts

There are many different types of cardiovascular workouts that readers can incorporate into their fitness routine. Below are some of the most effective types of cardio workouts:

Running

Running is an excellent form of cardiovascular exercise that requires no equipment and can be done almost anywhere. It's a high-impact activity that can help improve endurance, burn calories, and strengthen the muscles in the lower body.

Cycling

Cycling is another great form of cardiovascular exercise that can be done both indoors and outdoors. It's a low-impact activity that can help improve endurance, burn calories, and strengthen the muscles in the lower body.

Swimming

Swimming is a low-impact form of cardiovascular exercise that's great for people with joint pain or injuries. It's an excellent full-body workout that can help improve endurance, burn calories, and improve overall cardiovascular function.

HIIT, or high-intensity interval training, is a form of cardio that involves short bursts of intense exercise followed by periods of rest. It's a highly effective way to improve cardiovascular fitness, burn calories, and improve overall endurance.

Jumping Rope

Jumping rope is a simple yet effective form of cardiovascular exercise that can be done almost anywhere. It's a high-impact activity that can help improve endurance, burn calories, and strengthen the muscles in the lower body.

Incorporating Cardio Workouts into Your Fitness Routine

When incorporating cardio workouts into your fitness routine, it's essential to start slowly and gradually increase the intensity and duration of your workouts over time. It's also important to choose workouts that you enjoy and that fit your fitness level and personal preferences.

Aim to incorporate at least 30 minutes of moderate-intensity cardio exercise into your fitness routine most days of the week. You can also incorporate high-intensity cardio workouts into your routine a few times a week to help improve endurance and overall cardiovascular function.

Conclusion

In conclusion, cardiovascular fitness is essential for optimal health and fitness. Incorporating different types of cardio workouts into your fitness routine can help improve endurance, burn calories, and improve overall cardiovascular function. Whether it's running, cycling, swimming, HIIT, or jumping rope, there are many different types of cardio workouts to choose from. It's important to start slowly, choose workouts that you enjoy, and gradually increase the intensity and duration of your workouts over time.

Chapter 4: Strength Training

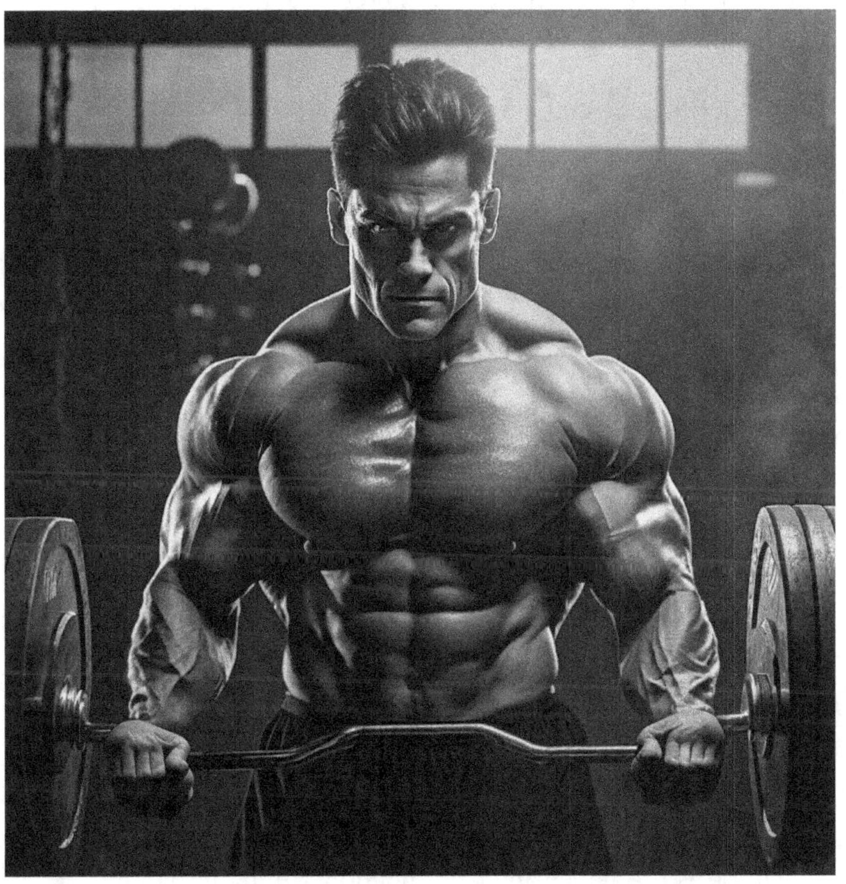

In this chapter, we'll discuss the benefits of strength training, provide instruction on proper form and technique, and offer various exercises and workouts for beginners to advanced levels.

Benefits of Strength Training

Strength training is a type of exercise that involves resistance or weight-bearing exercises that target the muscles. The benefits of strength training are numerous and include:

Increased Muscle Mass and Strength: Strength training helps increase muscle mass and strength, which can improve overall physical performance and help prevent injuries.

Improved Bone Health: Strength training can help improve bone density and reduce the risk of osteoporosis.

Increased Metabolic Rate: Strength training can help increase the body's metabolic rate, which can help burn more calories and improve overall weight management.

Improved Balance and Coordination: Strength training can help improve balance and coordination, which can help prevent falls and other injuries.

Proper Form and Technique

Proper form and technique are essential when it comes to strength training. Poor form can lead to injuries, and improper technique can limit the effectiveness of the exercise.

When performing strength training exercises, it's essential to:

Warm-Up: Before beginning any strength training exercises, it's important to warm-up and stretch to help prevent injuries.

Start with Light Weights: When starting with strength training, it's important to start with light weights and gradually increase the weight as your strength and endurance improves.

Use Proper Form: Proper form is essential when performing strength training exercises. It's important to maintain good posture, keep the core engaged, and avoid arching or rounding the back.

Breathe: Breathing is important when performing strength training exercises. It's essential to exhale when lifting the weight and inhale when returning to the starting position.

Exercises and Workouts

There are many different types of strength training exercises and workouts to choose from. Below are some of the most effective exercises and workouts for beginners to advanced levels:

Bodyweight Exercises: Bodyweight exercises are a great way to start with strength training. They don't require any equipment and can be done almost anywhere. Some effective bodyweight exercises include push-ups, squats, and lunges.

Resistance Band Exercises: Resistance band exercises are another great way to start with strength training. They're lightweight, portable, and can be done almost anywhere. Some effective resistance band exercises include bicep curls, tricep extensions, and chest presses.

Free Weight Exercises: Free weight exercises involve using dumbbells, barbells, or kettlebells to perform strength training exercises. They're more challenging than bodyweight exercises but can be more effective in building muscle mass and strength. Some effective free weight exercises include bench press, deadlifts, and squats.

Circuit Training: Circuit training involves performing a series of strength training exercises in a circuit with little rest in between. It's a highly effective way to improve overall strength and endurance. Some effective circuit training workouts include alternating lunges, push-ups, and kettlebell swings.

Conclusion

In conclusion, strength training is an essential component of overall fitness and health. It helps increase muscle mass and strength, improve bone health, increase the metabolic rate, and improve balance and coordination. When performing strength training exercises, it's important to use proper form and technique and to gradually increase the weight as your strength and endurance improves. Whether it's bodyweight exercises, resistance band exercises, free weight exercises, or circuit training, there are many different types of strength training exercises and workouts to choose from. It's important to choose exercises and workouts that fit your fitness level and personal preferences.

Chapter 5: Flexibility and Mobility

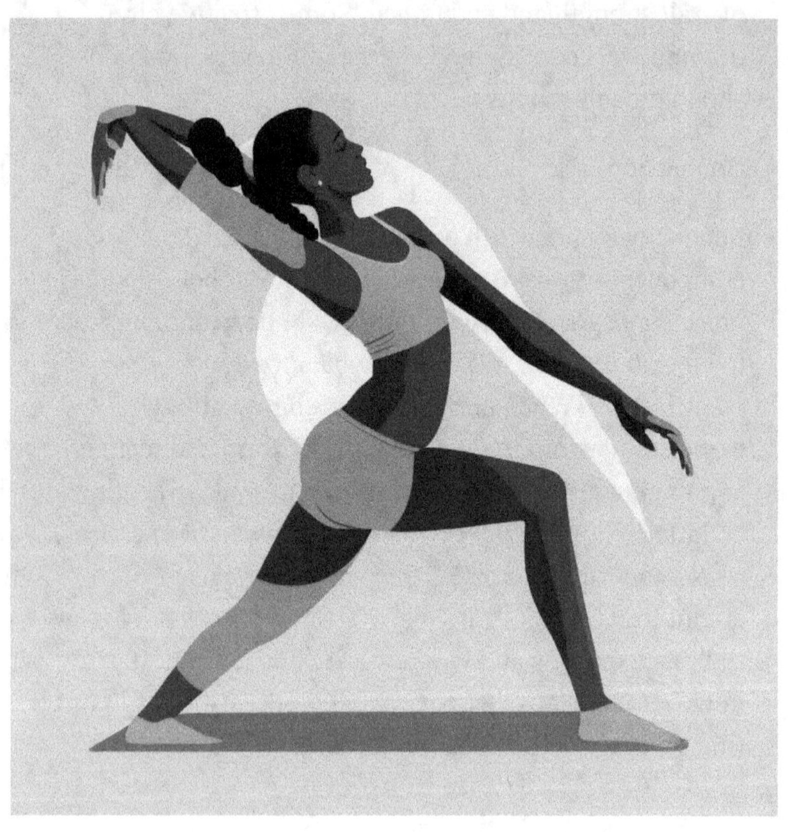

When it comes to achieving optimal fitness, many people focus solely on cardiovascular and strength training, often neglecting the importance of flexibility and mobility. However, flexibility and mobility are essential components of fitness, as they help improve range of motion, prevent injury, and maintain good posture. In this chapter, we will discuss the benefits of stretching, yoga, and other mobility exercises, and provide tips on how to incorporate them into your fitness routine.

Benefits of Flexibility and Mobility

Flexibility refers to the ability of a muscle or joint to move through its full range of motion, while mobility refers to the ability of a joint to move freely without restrictions or pain. Flexibility and mobility are crucial for maintaining good posture, preventing injury, and improving overall performance in other physical activities.

By regularly incorporating flexibility and mobility exercises into your fitness routine, you can:

Improve your range of motion: Stretching and mobility exercises can help you move more freely and with less pain, allowing you to perform better in other physical activities.

Reduce the risk of injury: Tight muscles and restricted joints can increase the risk of injury during physical activities, but stretching and mobility exercises can help reduce the risk of injury by improving your flexibility and mobility.

Maintain good posture: Poor posture can lead to muscle imbalances, back pain, and other issues, but stretching and mobility exercises can help improve your posture by correcting muscle imbalances and reducing tension in tight muscles.

Relieve stress and tension: Stretching and yoga can also have a calming effect on the mind and body, helping to relieve stress and tension.

Types of Flexibility and Mobility Exercises

There are many different types of flexibility and mobility exercises, including stretching, yoga, foam rolling, and dynamic mobility exercises. Each type of exercise offers unique benefits, and incorporating a variety of exercises into your fitness routine can help you achieve optimal results.

Stretching: Stretching involves holding a muscle in a lengthened position for a period of time to improve its flexibility. Static stretching, which involves holding a stretch without movement, is the most common type of stretching. Dynamic stretching, which involves moving through a range of motion, is also effective for improving flexibility and mobility.

Yoga: Yoga is a form of exercise that combines stretching, strength, and mindfulness. There are many different styles of yoga, each with its own unique benefits. Some styles, such as vinyasa or power yoga, are more vigorous and can help improve strength and cardiovascular fitness, while other styles, such as restorative or yin yoga, focus more on relaxation and stretching.

Foam Rolling: Foam rolling involves using a foam roller to apply pressure to different areas of the body, helping to release tension and improve mobility. Foam rolling can be especially effective for releasing tight muscles in the legs, back, and hips.

Dynamic Mobility Exercises: Dynamic mobility exercises involve moving through a range of motion, often in a controlled and deliberate manner. These exercises can help improve mobility and stability in the joints, and can be especially effective for warming up before exercise.

Incorporating Flexibility and Mobility Exercises into Your Fitness Routine

Incorporating flexibility and mobility exercises into your fitness routine can be simple and effective. Here are some tips to get you started:

Schedule time for stretching and mobility exercises: Just as you schedule time for cardio and strength training, it's important to make time for stretching and mobility exercises. Aim for at least 10-15 minutes of stretching and mobility exercises after each workout.

Start slowly: If you're new to stretching or mobility exercises, start slowly and gradually build up your flexibility and mobility over time. Don't push yourself too hard too quickly, as this can increase the risk of injury.

Mix it up: Incorporate a variety of stretching and mobility exercises.

In addition to stretching, yoga, and other mobility exercises, there are other methods you can use to improve your flexibility and mobility. These include using resistance bands, incorporating dynamic stretching into your warm-up routine, and practising specific exercises that target your problem areas.

Resistance bands are a great tool for improving flexibility and mobility, as they provide a gentle, gradual stretch that can help you improve your range of motion over time. You can use them to target specific muscle groups or incorporate them into your regular workouts for an extra challenge.

Dynamic stretching is a form of stretching that involves moving your body through a range of motions, rather than holding a static stretch. It helps to increase blood flow and warm up your muscles, making them more pliable and less prone to injury.

Some specific exercises that can improve your flexibility and mobility include hip flexor stretches, spine stretches, and calf stretches. These exercises help to improve your posture, reduce tension in your muscles, and increase your range of motion.

In this chapter, we will provide detailed instructions on how to use resistance bands, dynamic stretching techniques, and specific exercises to improve your flexibility and mobility. We will also include sample workouts that readers can follow to incorporate these techniques into their fitness routine.

By improving your flexibility and mobility, you can enhance your overall fitness and quality of life. You will be able to move more freely and easily, which can help you avoid injury, improve your posture, and even enhance your performance in other types of exercise.

In conclusion, flexibility and mobility are essential components of any fitness program. By incorporating stretching, yoga, foam rolling, mobility exercises, resistance bands, dynamic stretching, and specific exercises into your routine, you can improve your range of motion, reduce the risk of injury, and enhance your overall fitness and well-being.

Chapter 6: Recovery and Rest

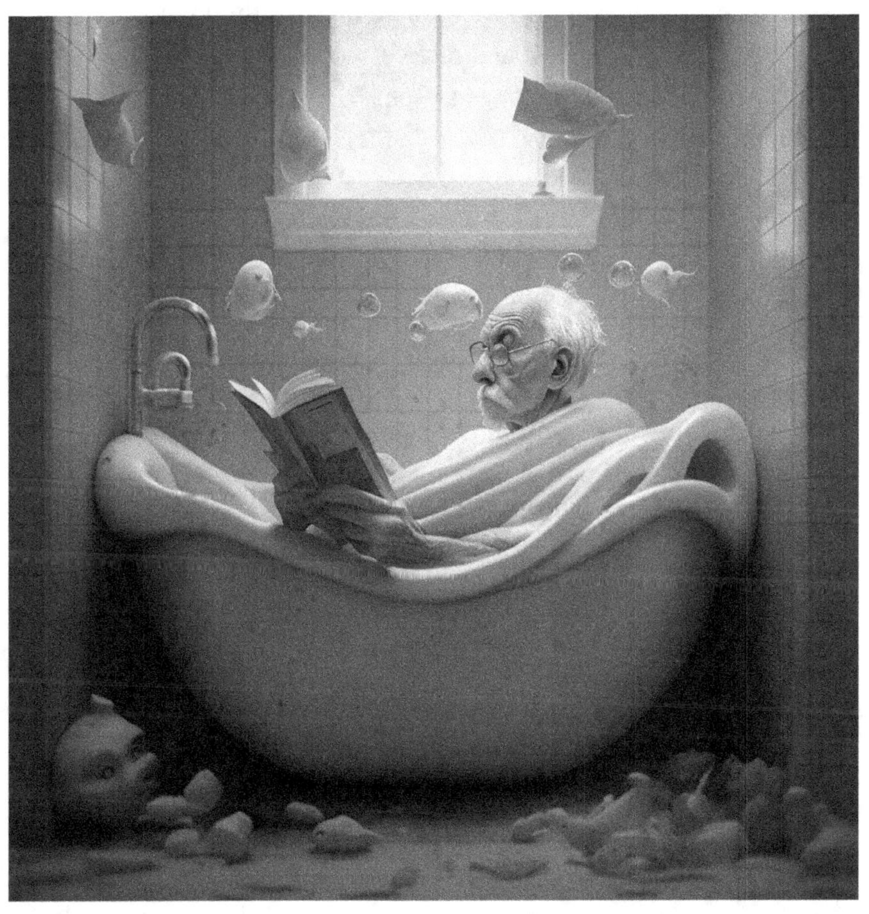

When it comes to getting fit, many people think that pushing themselves to their limits every day is the key to success. However, this mentality can actually do more harm than good. Rest and recovery are just as important as exercise when it comes to achieving optimal fitness and preventing injury.

In this chapter, we will discuss the importance of recovery and rest, and provide tips on how to properly recover from workouts and prevent injury.

Why Recovery and Rest Are Important

During exercise, your muscles undergo stress and strain, which causes small tears in the muscle fibres. These tears are necessary for muscle growth and strength gains, but they also require time to heal. Without proper recovery time, your muscles may not have the chance to fully repair themselves, which can lead to overuse injuries, fatigue, and a lack of progress.

Rest days are also important for mental and emotional health. Exercise can be a great way to relieve stress and improve mood, but constantly pushing yourself to the limit can also cause burnout and fatigue. Taking time to rest and recover can help you avoid these negative side effects and improve your overall well-being.

Tips for Proper Recovery

Here are some tips to help you recover properly after a workout:

Stretch: Stretching can help to prevent muscle soreness and tightness. Make sure to stretch both before and after your workout.

Hydrate: Drinking plenty of water can help to flush out toxins and reduce muscle soreness.

Get enough sleep: Sleep is essential for muscle recovery and overall health. Aim for 7-9 hours of sleep per night.

Incorporate active recovery: Active recovery involves engaging in low-intensity exercise, such as yoga or walking, to promote blood flow and reduce soreness.

Use foam rollers or massage balls: Foam rollers and massage balls can help to release tension and tightness in your muscles.

Preventing Injury

In addition to proper recovery, taking steps to prevent injury is also crucial. Here are some tips to help you stay injury-free:

Listen to your body: If you're feeling pain or discomfort, take a break or modify your workout.

Use proper form: Using proper form during exercise can help to prevent injuries.

Gradually increase intensity: Gradually increasing the intensity of your workouts can help to prevent overuse injuries.

Warm-up and cool-down: Warming up before exercise and cooling down afterwards can help to prevent injury and improve recovery.

Conclusion

Recovery and rest are just as important as exercise when it comes to achieving optimal fitness and preventing injury. By incorporating stretching, hydration, sleep, active recovery, and self-massage techniques into your routine, you can improve your recovery time and reduce the risk of injury. Remember to listen to your body, use proper form, gradually increase intensity, and warm-up and cool-down properly to stay healthy and injury-free.

Chapter 7: Motivation and Mindset

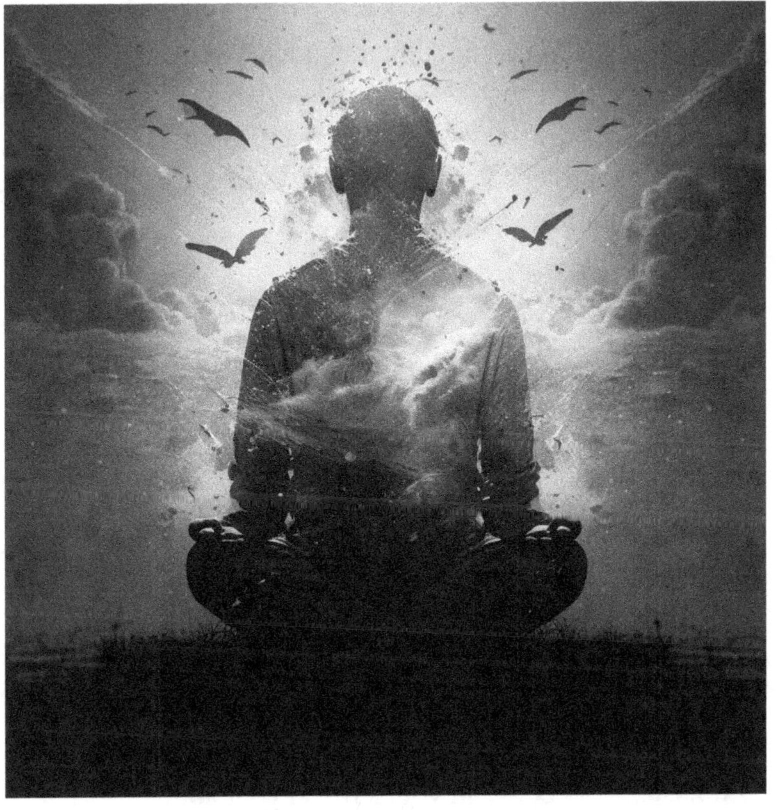

Getting started on a fitness journey can be tough, but it's even tougher to stay on track when things get tough. That's why having the right motivation and mindset is essential to achieving your fitness goals. In this chapter, we'll discuss the role of motivation and mindset in fitness and provide you with tips and strategies to help you stay motivated and positive.

The Importance of Motivation and Mindset

Motivation is what gets you started, but it's your mindset that keeps you going. Without the right mindset, even the most motivated person can struggle to stick to a fitness routine. A positive mindset can help you overcome obstacles, push through tough workouts, and stay committed to your goals.

There are many benefits to developing a positive mindset, including:

Increased self-confidence: When you have a positive mindset, you believe in yourself and your ability to achieve your goals.

Improved mental health: A positive mindset can reduce stress and anxiety, which can have a positive impact on your mental health.

Greater resilience: With a positive mindset, you're better able to bounce back from setbacks and stay motivated.

Tips for Staying Motivated and Positive

Set Realistic Goals: One of the best ways to stay motivated is to set realistic goals. Break your overall fitness goal into smaller, achievable goals that you can work towards each day or week.

Celebrate Your Progress: Celebrate your progress, no matter how small. Recognize your achievements, and don't be too hard on yourself if you slip up. Remember that every setback is an opportunity to learn and grow.

Find an Accountability Partner: Having an accountability partner can be a great way to stay motivated. Find a friend or family member who shares your fitness goals and can help keep you accountable.

Mix Up Your Routine: Doing the same workout every day can quickly become boring. Mix up your routine with different types of workouts, and challenge yourself to try new things.

Focus on the Positive: Instead of focusing on what you can't do, focus on what you can do. Celebrate your strengths, and work on improving your weaknesses.

Practice Self-Care: Taking care of yourself is essential for staying motivated and positive. Get enough sleep, eat a healthy diet, and make time for relaxation and self-care.

Developing a positive mindset takes time and practice, but it's well worth the effort. By staying motivated and positive, you can achieve your fitness goals and enjoy a happier, healthier life.

Chapter 8: Home Workouts

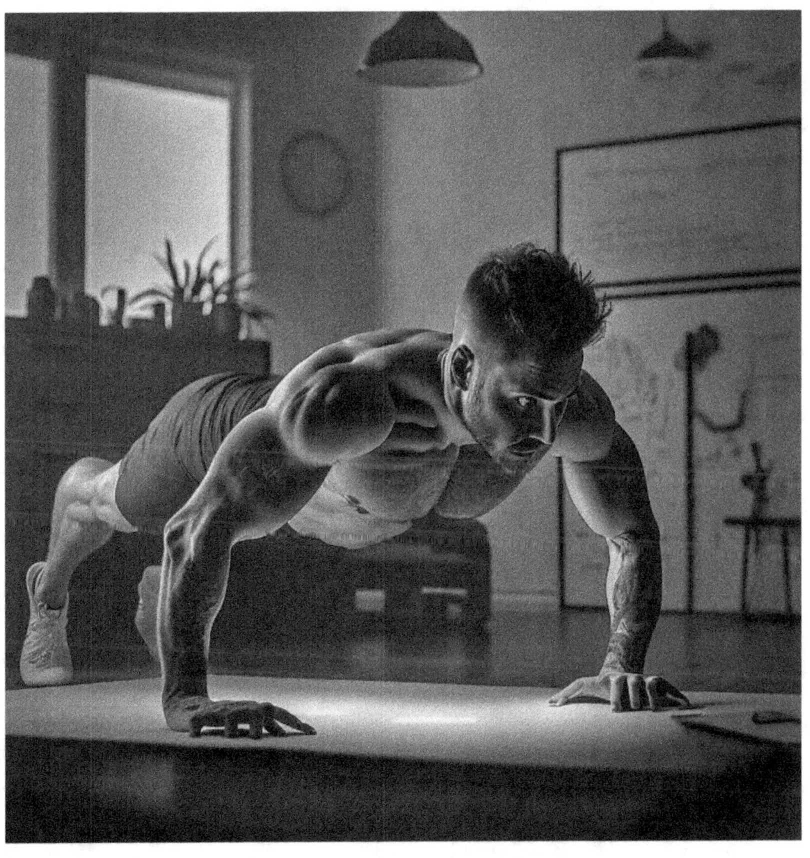

For many people, finding the time and resources to go to a gym can be a challenge. However, with a little creativity and some simple equipment, it's possible to get a great workout in the comfort of your own home. In this chapter, we'll discuss tips and strategies for working out at home with limited equipment.

Bodyweight Exercises

One of the easiest and most effective ways to work out at home is by using your own bodyweight. Bodyweight exercises can be done anywhere and require no equipment. They also offer a variety of benefits, including improved strength, flexibility, and endurance.

Some examples of bodyweight exercises include push-ups, squats, lunges, and planks. These exercises can be modified to suit your fitness level and can be combined into a full-body workout.

At-Home Equipment

While bodyweight exercises can be effective, adding some basic equipment can help you take your workouts to the next level. Some examples of at-home equipment include resistance bands, dumbbells, and exercise balls.

Resistance bands are lightweight and portable, making them ideal for at-home workouts. They can be used for a variety of exercises, including bicep curls, tricep extensions, and rows. Dumbbells are also versatile and can be used for a variety of exercises, including squats, lunges, and chest presses. Exercise balls can be used for core-strengthening exercises, such as planks and crunches.

Creating a Home Gym

If you have the space and budget, creating a home gym can be a great investment. This can be as simple as setting up a designated workout area with a mat and some equipment, or as elaborate as outfitting a dedicated room with a full range of equipment.

When setting up a home gym, it's important to consider your fitness goals and choose equipment accordingly. Some basic pieces of equipment to consider include a bench, barbells, dumbbells, a treadmill or elliptical machine, and a pull-up bar.

Workout Programs

Having a workout program can help you stay on track and achieve your fitness goals. There are many home workout programs available online, ranging from beginner to advanced levels.

When choosing a workout program, it's important to consider your fitness level, time commitment, and equipment availability. Many programs can be modified to suit your needs, and it's important to listen to your body and make adjustments as needed.

Conclusion

Working out at home can be a convenient and effective way to stay fit and healthy. Whether you're using bodyweight exercises, at-home equipment, or setting up a home gym, there are many options available to suit your needs. With a little motivation and dedication, you can achieve your fitness goals from the comfort of your own home.

Chapter 9: Staying Active

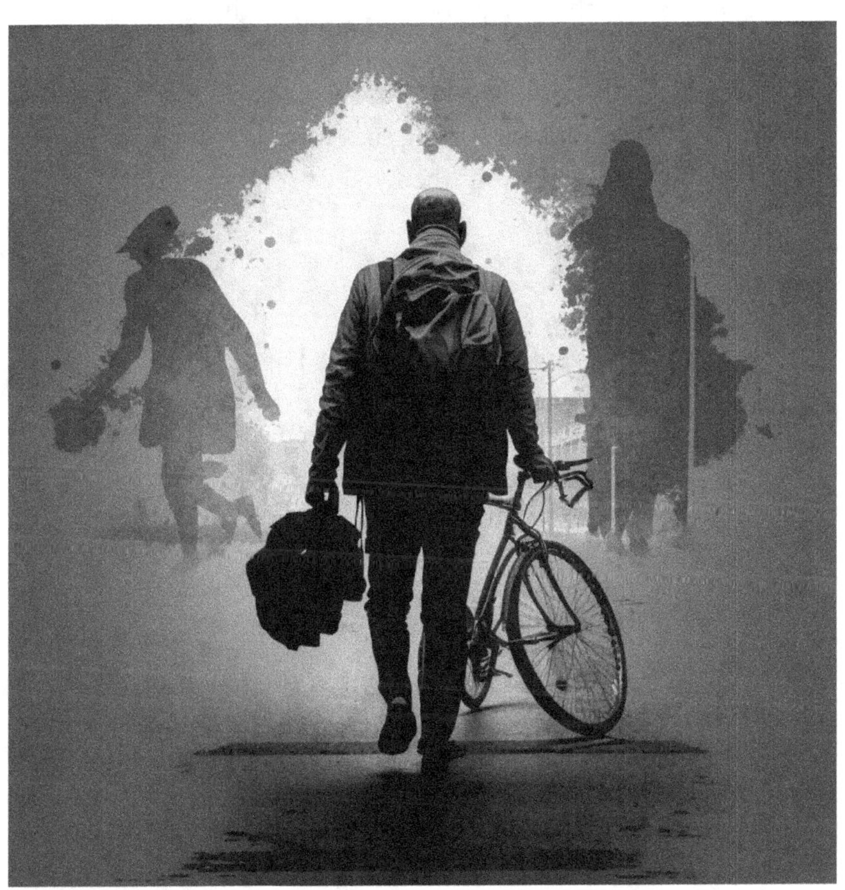

Exercise is important, but staying active throughout the day is just as crucial for your overall health and fitness. Incorporating physical activity into your daily life can help you maintain a healthy weight, reduce the risk of chronic diseases, improve mood, and boost energy levels. In this chapter, we'll discuss ways to stay active throughout the day, even when you can't hit the gym.

Take the Stairs

Taking the stairs is an easy way to get some extra physical activity into your day. Instead of taking the elevator, opt for the stairs whenever possible. Even taking the stairs for just a few flights can help boost your heart rate and burn some extra calories.

Go for a Walk

Walking is one of the easiest and most accessible forms of physical activity. Take a walk during your lunch break, walk to the store instead of driving, or go for an after-dinner stroll. Walking can help improve cardiovascular health, reduce stress levels, and boost mood.

Stand Up and Stretch

Sitting for long periods of time can be detrimental to your health, but taking breaks to stand up and stretch can help counteract some of the negative effects of sitting. Set a timer on your phone or computer to remind you to stand up and stretch every hour or so.

Desk Exercises

There are plenty of exercises you can do at your desk to stay active throughout the day. Try doing some squats, lunges, or calf raises while you're on the phone, or do some shoulder shrugs to relieve tension in your upper back and neck.

Dance

Dancing is a fun and easy way to get your heart rate up and burn some extra calories. Turn on some music and dance around your living room, or take a dance class with friends.

Gardening

Gardening is a great way to stay active and enjoy the outdoors. Whether you have a large backyard or just a few potted plants on your balcony, tending to your garden can help improve flexibility, strength, and endurance.

Household Chores

Household chores like vacuuming, sweeping, and doing laundry can all help you stay active throughout the day. Make a game out of it by timing yourself and trying to beat your previous record.

Active Commuting

If you live close enough to work, consider biking or walking instead of driving. Not only will you get some extra physical activity, but you'll also save money on gas and reduce your carbon footprint.

Take Active Breaks

Instead of taking coffee or snack breaks, take active breaks. Go for a quick walk around the block, do some stretching, or try some desk exercises.

Stand Up Meetings

Instead of sitting in a conference room for meetings, suggest standing up or even going for a walk while discussing business. This can help boost creativity and productivity, as well as provide some physical activity.

Incorporating physical activity into your daily life doesn't have to be complicated or time-consuming. By

making small changes to your routine, you can improve
your overall health and fitness.

Chapter 10: Advanced Fitness

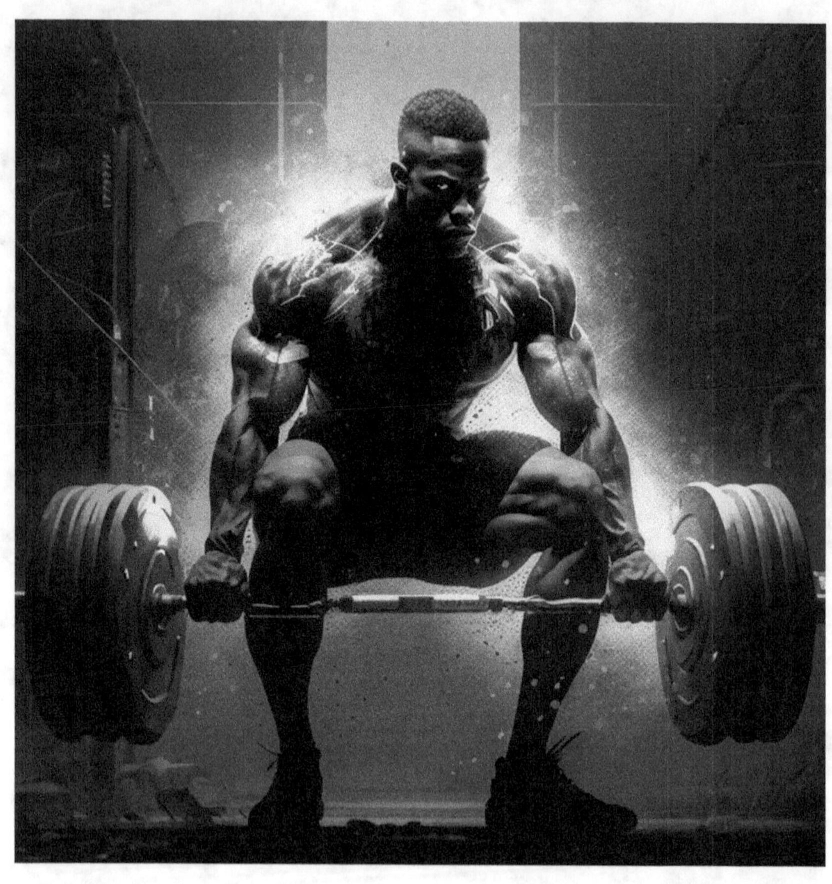

Congratulations on making it to the final chapter of this fitness guide! If you're reading this, it's likely that you have made significant progress in your fitness journey and are now looking for more advanced tips and strategies to take your fitness to the next level. This chapter will focus on advanced fitness, including tips for training for a specific sport or event, bodybuilding, and powerlifting.

Training for a Specific Sport or Event

If you're looking to take your fitness to the next level, training for a specific sport or event can be a great way to do so. Whether it's running a marathon, competing in a triathlon, or playing a specific sport, training for a specific event can help you stay focused and motivated. Here are some tips for training for a specific sport or event:

Set specific goals: When training for a specific sport or event, it's important to set specific goals. For example, if you're training for a marathon, set a goal time that you want to achieve.

Develop a training plan: A training plan will help you stay organised and ensure that you're progressing toward your goals. Your training plan should include workouts that are specific to the sport or event that you're training for.

Incorporate cross-training: Cross-training can help you build strength and improve your overall fitness. Incorporate activities such as swimming, cycling, or weight lifting into your training plan.

Bodybuilding

If you're looking to build muscle and increase your overall strength, bodybuilding may be the right choice for you. Bodybuilding involves lifting heavy weights and focusing on building specific muscle groups. Here are some tips for bodybuilding:

Lift heavy weights: To build muscle, you need to lift heavy weights. Focus on lifting weights that are challenging but still allow you to maintain proper form.

Eat a high-protein diet: Protein is essential for building muscle. Make sure you're eating enough protein to support muscle growth.

Focus on specific muscle groups: To maximise muscle growth, focus on specific muscle groups during each workout. For example, one day you may focus on your chest and triceps, and the next day you may focus on your back and biceps.

Powerlifting

Powerlifting is a strength sport that involves lifting as much weight as possible for three main lifts: squat, bench press, and deadlift. If you're looking to increase your overall strength, powerlifting may be the right choice for you. Here are some tips for powerlifting:

Focus on the main lifts: The squat, bench press, and deadlift are the main lifts in powerlifting. Make sure you're focusing on these lifts during your workouts.

Lift heavy weights: To get stronger, you need to lift heavy weights. Make sure you're challenging yourself with each workout.

Incorporate assistance exercises: Assistance exercises such as lunges, pull-ups, and dips can help you build strength and improve your overall fitness.

Conclusion

Congratulations on completing this fitness guide! Whether you're a beginner or an advanced fitness enthusiast, this guide has provided you with tips and strategies for achieving your fitness goals. Remember, fitness is a journey, not a destination. Keep working hard, stay motivated, and most importantly, enjoy the process.

9 798390 501283